Easy and Tasty

Keto Ideas

Recipes for rapid weight loss and healthier eating habits

Charlotte Willis

TABLE OF CONTENTS

3

content within this book has been derived from various sources. Please consult a licensed professional before attempting any techniques outlined in this book. By reading this document, the reader agrees that under no circumstances is the author responsible for any losses, 5 direct or indirect, which are incurred as a result of the use of information contained within this document, including, but not limited to, — errors, omissions, or inaccuracies.

BREAKFAST

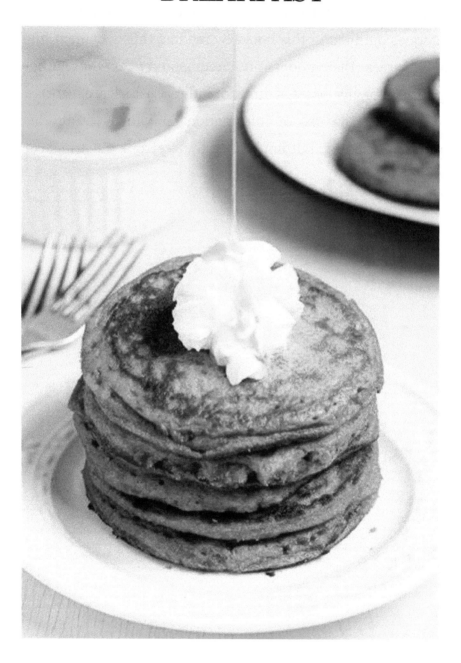

Coconut Berries Bowls

Servings: 4

Cooking Time: 0 minutes

Ingredients

- 1 cup blackberries
- 1 cup strawberries
- 1 cup raspberries1 tablespoon lime juice
- ¼ cup almonds, cubed
- 2 teaspoons coconut oil, melted

Directions:

1. In a bowl, combine the strawberries with the blackberries and the rest of the ingredients, toss, divide into small bowls, and serve breakfast.

Nutrition Info:

Calories 200, fat 7.5, fiber 4, carbs 5.7, protein 8

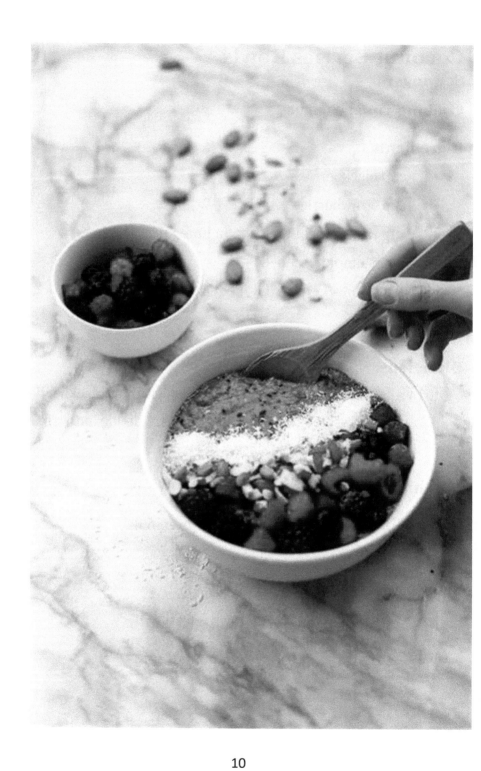

Delicious Pumpkin Pancakes

Servings: 6

Cooking Time: 15 minutes

Ingredients

- 1-ounce egg white protein
- 2 ounces hazelnut flour
- 2 ounces flax seeds, ground
- 1 teaspoon baking powder
- 1 cup coconut cream
- 1 tablespoon chai masala
- 1 teaspoon vanilla extract
- ½ cup pumpkin puree
- 3 eggs
- 5 drops stevia
- 1 tablespoon swerve
- 1 teaspoon coconut oil

Directions:

1. In a bowl, mix flax seeds with hazelnut flour, egg white protein, baking powder and chai masala and stir.
2. In another bowl, mix coconut cream with vanilla extract, pumpkin puree, eggs, stevia and swerve and stir well.
3. Combine the 2 mixtures and stir well.

4. Heat up a pan. With the oil over medium-high heat, pour 1/6 of the batter, spread into a circle, cover, reduce heat to low, cook for 3 minutes on each side and transfer to a plate.

5. Repeat this and serve your pumpkin pancakes right away.

6. Enjoy!

Nutrition Info: calories 400, fat 23, fiber 4, carbs 5, protein 21

Spicy Egg Muffins with Bacon & Cheese

Servings: 6

Cooking Time: 30 minutes

Ingredients

- 12 eggs
- ¼ cup of coconut milk
- Salt and black pepper to taste
- 1 cup grated cheddar cheese
- 12 slices bacon
- 4 jalapeño peppers, seeded and minced

Directions:

1. Preheat oven to 370° F.

2. Crack the eggs and whisk with coconut milk until combined. Season with salt and pepper, and evenly stir in the cheddar cheese.

3. Line all of the holes of a muffin tin with a bacon slice and fill each with the egg mixture two-thirds way up. Top with the jalapeno peppers and bake in the oven for 18 to 20 minutes or until puffed and golden. Remove, allow cooling for a few minutes, and serve with arugula salad.

Nutrition Info (Per Serving): Kcal 302, Fat 23.7g, Net Carbs 3.2g, Protein 20g

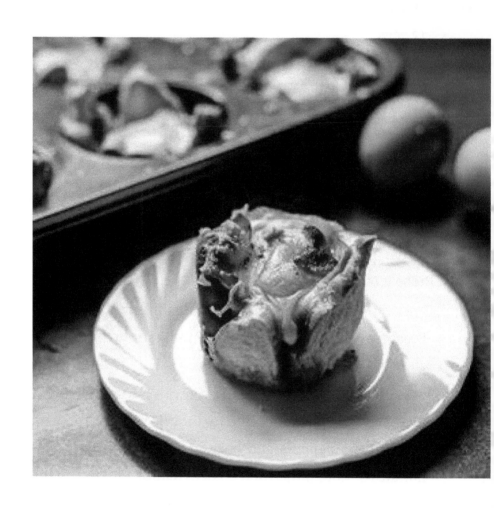

Simple Smoothie Bowl

Servings: 1

Cooking Time: 0 minutes

Ingredients

- 2 ice cubes
- 1 tablespoon coconut oil
- 2 tablespoons heavy cream
- 1 cup spinach
- ½ cup almond milk
- 1 teaspoon protein powder
- 4 raspberries
- 1 tablespoon coconut, shredded
- 4 walnuts
- 1 teaspoon chia seeds

Directions:

1. In your blender, mix milk with spinach, cream, ice, protein powder and coconut oil, blend well and transfer to a bowl.

2. Top your bowl with raspberries, coconut, walnuts and chia seeds and serve.

3. Enjoy!

Nutrition Info: calories 450, fat 34, fiber 4, carbs 4, protein 35

Chocolate Crepes with Caramel Cream

Servings: 4

Cooking Time: 35 minutes

Ingredients

- 4 tbsp coconut flour
- 4 tbsp unsweetened cocoa powder
- ½ tsp baking powder
- 4 egg whites
- ½ cup + 4 tbsp flax milk
- 2 tbsp erythritol
- 2 tbsp olive oil

- Caramel Cream:
- ½ cup salted butter
- 4 tbsp swerve brown sugar
- 1 tsp vanilla extract
- 1 cup heavy cream

Directions:

1. In a bowl, mix the coconut flour, cocoa powder, and baking powder together. Set aside.
1. 2. In another bowl, whisk the egg whites, ½ cup flax milk, erythritol, and olive oil. Pour the wet ingredients now into the dry ingredients, and whisk until smooth.

2. Set a skillet over medium heat, grease with cooking spray, and pour in a ladleful of the batter. Swirl the pan quickly to spread the dough all around the skillet and cook the crepe for 2-minutes.

3. When it is firm enough to touch and cooked through, slide the crepe into a flat plate. Wipe the pan with a napkin and continue cooking until the remaining batter has finished.

4. Put the butter and brown sugar in a pot and melt the butter over medium heat while stirring continually. Keep cooking for 4 minutes after the butter has melted; be careful not to burn.

5. Stir in the cream, reduce the heat to low, and let the sauce simmer for

6. 10 minutes while stirring continually. Turn the heat off and stir into the vanilla extract. Once the crepes are ready, drizzle the caramel sauce over them, and serve with a cup of coffee.

Nutrition Info (Per Serving): Kcal 330, Fat 21g, Net Carbs 5.1g, Protein 11g

Amazing Breakfast Hash

Servings: 2

Cooking Time: 16 minutes

Ingredients

- 1 tablespoon coconut oil
- 2 garlic cloves, minced
- ½ cup beef stock
- Salt and black pepper to the taste
- 1 yellow onion, chopped
- 2 cups corned beef, chopped
- 1 pound radishes, cut in quarters

Directions:

1. Heat up a pan. Oil over medium-high heat, add some onion, stir and cook for 4 minutes.

2. Add radishes, stir and cook for 5 minutes.

3. Add some garlic, stir and cook for 1 minute more.

4. Add stock, beef, salt and pepper, stir, cook for 5 minutes, take off the heat and serve.

5. Enjoy!

Nutrition Info: calories 240, fat 7, fiber 3, carbs 12, protein 8

BRUNCH

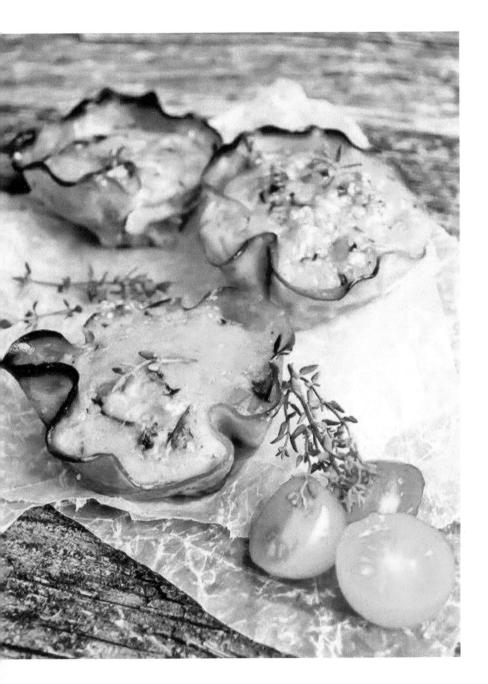

Brussels Sprouts Delight

Servings: 3

Cooking Time: 12 minutes

Ingredients

- 3 eggs
- Salt and black pepper to the taste
- 1 tablespoon ghee, melted
- 2 shallots, minced
- 2 garlic cloves, minced
- 12 ounces Brussels sprouts, thinly sliced
- 2 ounces bacon, chopped
- 1 and ½ tablespoons apple cider vinegar

Directions:

1. Heat up a pan over medium heat. Add bacon, stir, cook until it's crispy, transfer to a plate and leave aside for now.

2. Heat up the pan over medium heat. Add shallots, garlic. Stir and cook for 30 seconds.

3. Add Brussels sprouts, salt, pepper and apple cider vinegar, stir and cook for 5 minutes.

4. Return bacon to pan, stir and cook for 5 minutes more.

5. Add ghee, stir and make a hole in the center.

6. Crack eggs into the pan, cook until they are done and serve right away.

7. Enjoy!

Nutrition Info: calories 240, fat 7, fiber 4, carbs 7, protein 12

Pesto Bread Twists

Servings: 6

Cooking Time: 35 minutes

Ingredients

- 1 tbsp flax seed powder, + 3 tbsp water
- 1½ cups grated mozzarella
- 4 tbsp coconut flour
- ½ cup almond flour
- 1 tsp baking powder
- 5 tbsp butter
- 2 oz pesto

Directions:

1. For flax egg, mix flax seed powder with water in a bowl and soak for 5 minutes.

2. Preheat the oven to 350 F; line a baking sheet with parchment paper.

3. In a bowl, combine coconut flour, almond flour, salt, and baking powder.

4. Melt butter and cheese in a skillet and stir in the flax egg. Mix in flour mixture until a firm dough forms.

5. Divide the mixture between 2 parchment papers, then use a rolling pin to flatten out the dough of about an inch's thickness. Remove the parchment paper on top and spread pesto all over the dough.

6. Cut the dough into strips, twist each piece, and place it on the baking sheet.

7. Brush with olive oil and bake for -20 minutes until golden brown.

Nutrition Info (Per Serving): Cal 206; Net Carbs 3g; Fat 17g; Protein 8g

Ham, Cheese, & Egg Cups

Servings: 6

Cooking Time: 30 minutes

Ingredients

- 6 thin slices of ham
- 1 teaspoon mustard
- 6 eggs
- 4 ounces cream cheese
- 1/2 teaspoon red pepper flakes, crushed Garlic
- salt and ground black pepper, to taste
- 6 ounces Colby cheese, shredded
- 2 tablespoons green onions, chopped

Directions:

1. Spritz a muffin tin with nonstick cooking spray. Place the ham slices over each muffin cup and gently press down until a cup shape forms.

2. In a mixing dish, whisk the mustard, eggs, cream cheese, red pepper, garlic salt, and black pepper.

3. Divide the egg mixture between the cups. Top with the shredded Colby cheese. Bake in the preheated oven at 0 degrees F for approximately 25 minutes.

4. Transfer the muffin tin to a wire rack before serving. Garnish with green onions and serve. Bon appétit!

Nutrition Info (Per Serving): 258 Calories; 19.1g Fat; 2.8g Carbs; 17.5g Protein; 0.2g Fiber

Bresaola & Mozzarella Scrambled Eggs

Servings: 3

Cooking Time: 15 minutes

Ingredients

- 6 eggs
- A bunch of chives, chopped
- 2 ounces mozzarella cheese
- 1 tbsp butter
- 1 tbsp water
- 4 thin slices of bresaola
- Salt and black pepper, to taste

Directions:

1. Crack the eggs in a bowl, whisk in water, salt and pepper. Melt the butter in a skillet and cook the eggs, constantly stirring for 30 seconds.
2. Spread bresaola slices over and top with mozzarella. Stir and cook for 3 minutes until the omelet is set. Sprinkle with fresh chives and serve.

Nutrition Info (Per Serving): Cal 224; Net Carbs 2.2g; Fat 15g; Protein 19g

Avocado Pate with Flaxseed Toasts

Servings: 4

Cooking Time: 5 minutes

Ingredients

- 1/2 cup flaxseed meal
- 1 pinch salt

- For the Avocado pate:
- 3 ripe avocado, chopped
- 4 tbsp Greek yogurt
- 2 tbsp chopped green onions
- 1 lemon, zested and juiced
- Black pepper to taste
- Smoked paprika to garnish

Directions:

1. For the flaxseed toasts:
2. Preheat oven to 350° F. Place a skillet over medium heat. Mix in flaxseed meal, 1/4 cup water, and salt and mix continually to form the dough into a ball.
3. Place the dough between parchment papers, put on a flat surface, and flatten thinly with a rolling pin.
4. Remove the papers and cut the pastry into tortilla chips.

5. Place on a baking sheet and bake for 8- 12 minutes or until crispy.

6. In a bowl, mix avocado, yogurt, green onions, lemon zest, juice, and black pepper until evenly combined.

7. Spread the paste on the toasts and garnish with paprika. Serve immediately.

Nutrition Info (Per Serving): Cal 364; Net Carbs 4g, Fat 31g, Protein 7.4g

SOUP AND STEWS

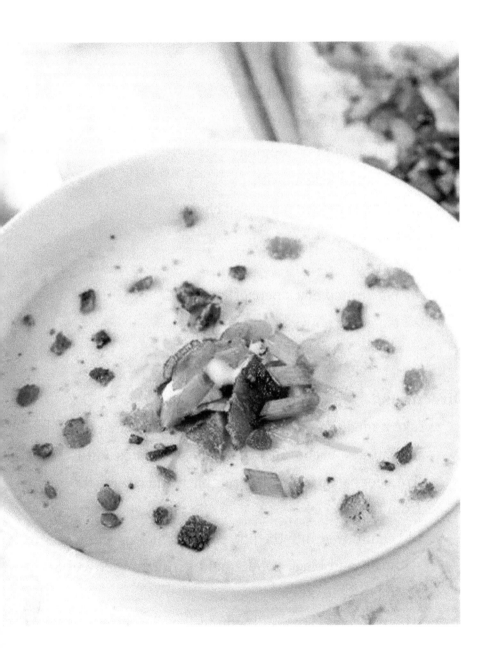

Cheese and Cauliflower Soup

Servings: 2

Cooking Time: 15 minutes

Ingredients

- 4 ounce chopped cauliflower
- 2 slices of turkey bacon
- 1 ¾ tbsp whipped topping
- 1 1/2 cups chicken broth
- 4-ounce shredded parmesan cheese
- Seasoning:
- ½ tsp salt
- ½ tsp ground black pepper
- ¼ tsp garlic powder

Directions:

1. Take a medium pot, place it over medium-high heat, then add turkey bacon and cook for 5 minutes until crispy. Transfer bacon to a plate, crumble it and reserve the grease from the pot.

2. Add cauliflower into the pot, pour in chicken broth, season with salt and black pepper, add garlic powder and bring the mixture to boil.

3. Then lower heat to medium-low level and simmer cauliflower for 5 to 7 minutes until tender.

4. Remove pot from the heat, puree the mixture with an immersion blender, then add cheese and whipped topping and stir until well combined. Ladle soup into bowls, top with bacon and serve.

Nutrition Info: 123.5 Calories; 9.3 g Fats; 4.5 g Protein; 1.2 g Net Carb; 0.4 g Fiber;

Mushroom Soup

Servings: 4

Cooking Time: 20 minutes

Ingredients

- 3 tablespoons unsalted butter
- 1 scallion, sliced
- 1 garlic clove, crushed
- 5 cups fresh mushrooms, sliced
- 2 cups homemade vegetable broth
- Salt and ground black pepper, as required
- 1 cup heavy cream

Directions:

1. Melt the butter in a large pan over medium heat and sauté the scallion and garlic for about 2-3 minutes.
2. Add the mushrooms and stir fry for about 5 minutes.
3. Stir in the broth and bring to a boil.
4. Cook for about 5 minutes.
5. Remove from the heat and blend the soup until smooth.
6. Return the pan over medium heat.
7. Stir in the cream, salt, and black pepper and cook for about 2-3 minutes, stirring continuously.
8. Serve hot.

Nutrition Info (Per Serving): Calories: 220; Net Casouprbs: 3.7g; Carbohydrate: 4.7g; Fiber: 1g; Protein: 6g; Fat: 20.7g; Sugar: 2g; Sodium: 499mg

Keto Cabbage Soup

Preparation Time: 10 minutes

Cooking Time: 30 minutes

Servings: 6

Ingredients:

- 1/4 cup onion, diced
- 1 clove garlic, minced
- 1 tsp. cumin
- 1 head cabbage, chopped
- 1 1/4 cup canned diced tomatoes
- 5 oz. canned green chilis
- 4 cups vegetable stock
- Salt and pepper to taste

Directions:

1. Heat a heavy stockpot over medium-high heat. Add the onions and sauté for 5- 7 minutes more. Add the garlic and sauté for one more minute.

2. Bring this to a low simmer and cook until the vegetables are tender about 30 minutes. And add water, if necessary, during cooking.

3. Transfer to serving bowls and serve hot.

Nutrition:

Calories: 131 Fat: 4.3g Fiber: 5.9g Carbohydrates: 1.2 g Protein: 5.1

Mixed Vegetable Stew

Preparation Time: 15 minutes

Cooking Time: 30 minutes

Servings: 6

Ingredients:

- 1 turnip, cut into bite-size pieces
- 1 onion, chopped
- 6 stalks celery, diced
- 1 carrot, sliced
- 15 oz. pumpkin puree
- lb. green beans frozen or fresh
- 8 cups chicken stock
- cups of water
- 1 Tbsp. fresh basil, chopped
- 1/4 tsp. thyme leaves
- 1/8 tsp. rubbed sage
- Salt to taste
- 1 lb. fresh spinach, chopped

Directions:

1. Put all the ingredients, excluding the spinach, into a heavy stockpot.

2. Bring to a low simmer and cook until the vegetables are tender about 30 minutes. Add water, if necessary, during cooking.

3. Add the spinach and stir until it's wilted about 5 minutes. Transfer to serving bowls and serve hot.

Nutrition:

Calories: 198 Fat: 6.4g Fiber: 11.3g Carbohydrates: 2.5 g Protein: 8.2g

Vegetarian Green Chili

Preparation Time: 15 minutes

Cooking Time: 20 minutes

Servings: 6

Ingredients:

- 3 tomatillos, sliced
- 3 jalapeno peppers, seeded and chopped
- 2 New Mexico green chili peppers, seeded and chopped
- 6 cloves garlic, minced
- 1 tomato, chopped
- 3 cups vegetable stock
- 2 tsp. cumin
- Salt and pepper to taste

Directions:

1. Put the tomatillos, jalapenos, New Mexico chilis, garlic, chicken stock, and tomato into a heavy stockpot.

2. Add the cumin, salt, and pepper on top of the meat.

3. Simmer and cook until fragrant, about 20 minutes. Add water, if necessary, during cooking.

4. Puree the soup until smooth.

5. Transfer the chili to serving bowls and serve hot, garnished with chopped fresh cilantro.

Nutrition:

Calories: 201 Fat: 6.1g Fiber: 11.2g Carbohydrates: 2.1 g Protein: 5.1g

MAIN

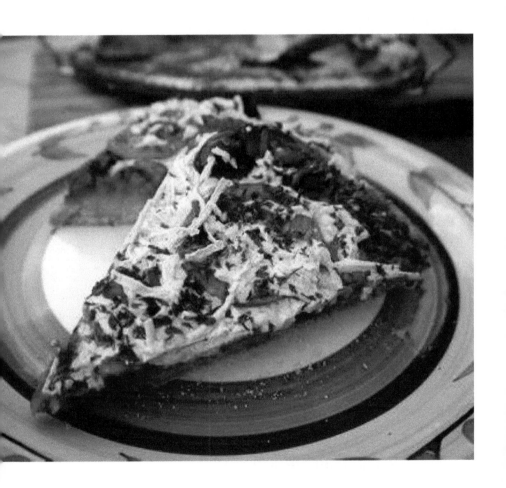

Mushroom Risotto

Servings: 4

Preparation Time: 5 minutes

Cooking Time: 10 minutes

Ingredients:

- Cauliflower -riced: 4 ½ cups
- Coconut oil: 3 tablespoon
- Portabello mushrooms -thinly sliced: 1 lb.
- White mushrooms -thinly sliced: 1 lb.
- Shallots -diced: 2
- Organic vegetable broth: ¼ cup
- Sea salt: to taste
- Ground black pepper: to taste
- Chives -finely chopped: 3 tablespoon
- Butter: 4 tablespoon
- Parmesan cheese -freshly grated: 1/3 cup

Directions:

1. Heat 2 tbsps. oil in a saucepan and sauté the mushrooms for 3 minutes until softened.
2. Transfer into a bowl.
3. Add the rest of the oil to the skillet and sauté the shallots in it for a minute.
4. Add in the cauliflower rice, cooking for 2 minutes.

5. Pour in the broth and cook until the broth is absorbed for 5 minutes.

6. Remove from the flame and mix in the rest of the ingredients.

Nutrition Value:

264 Cal, 17.1 g total fat, 13.5 g carbs, 5.1 g fiber, 11.9 g protein.

Spaghetti Squash Bowls with Egg & Avocado

Servings: 2

Preparation Time: 10 minutes

Cooking Time: 60 minutes

Ingredients:

- Spaghetti squash -halved, seeds discarded: 1
- Ripe Haas avocado -diced: 1
- Pepper Jack cheese -shredded: 4 oz.
- Eggs: 2
- Extra-virgin olive oil: 2 tablespoon
- Salt and pepper: to taste
- Sriracha: 2 teaspoon

Directions:

1. Season the squash with salt and pepper and drizzle oil on each.

2. Roast the squash, cut side down in an oven preheated to 400 degrees Fahrenheit for 40 minutes.

3. Leave to cool for 15 minutes, cut side up.

4. Gently scrape the squash flesh into noodles within the skin itself and mix it with the avocado and 2 oz cheese.

5. Crack an egg into each half of the squash and sprinkle the rest of the cheese over.

6. Bake for 20 minutes at 425 degrees Fahrenheit.

Nutrition Value:

559 Cal, 46 g total fat, 19 g carbs, 22 g protein.

Greek-style Pizza

Servings: 4

Cooking Time: 30 minutes

Ingredients

- ½ cup almond flour
- ¼ tsp salt
- 2 tbsp ground psyllium husk
- 1 tbsp olive oil
- ¼ tsp red chili flakes
- ¼ tsp dried Greek seasoning
- 1 cup crumbled feta cheese
- 3 sliced plum tomatoes
- 6 Kalamata olives, chopped
- 5 basil leaves, chopped

Directions:

1. Preheat the oven to 390° F, then line a baking sheet with parchment paper.

2. In a bowl, mix almond flour, salt, psyllium powder, olive oil, and a cup of lukewarm water until dough forms.

3. Spread the mixture on the pizza pan and bake for 10 minutes.

4. Sprinkle the red chili flakes and Greek seasoning on the crust and top with the feta cheese.

5. Arrange the tomatoes and olives on top. Bake for 10 minutes.

6. Garnish pizza with basil, slice and serve warm.

Nutrition Info (Per Serving): Cal 276; Net Carbs 4.5g; Fats 12g; Protein 8g

Zucchini Noodle Carbonara

Servings: 2

Cooking Time: 10 minutes

Ingredients

- 2 large zucchini
- 1 large egg
- 1 egg yolk
- ¼ cup grated cheddar cheese
- 3 slices of turkey bacon, diced

Seasoning:

- 1/4 tsp sea salt
- 1/2 tsp fresh ground black pepper

Directions:

1. Prepare zucchini noodles, and for this, cut off the bottom and top of zucchini and then use a spiralizer to convert them into noodles.

2. Take a baking sheet, line it with a paper towel, then lay the zucchini noodles on them, sprinkle with salt, and let sit for 5 minutes. Then wrap zucchini noodles in a cheesecloth and squeeze well to remove its liquid as much as possible and set aside until required. Prepare the sauce and for this, crack the egg in a bowl, add egg yolk and cheese and whisk until well combined. Take a skillet pan, place it over medium heat, add bacon slices, and cook for 3 to 5 minutes

until crispy. Then add zucchini noodles and cook for 3 minutes until warmed through. Switch heat to a low level, pour in egg mixture, stir well and remove the pan from heat. Stir the zucchini noodle until the egg is just cooked and then sprinkle with black pepper

3. Serve.

Nutrition Info: 114 Calories; 7 g Fats; 8 g Protein; 1.5 g Net Carb; 1.5 g Fiber

Mexicana Cauliflower Rice

Servings: 3

Preparation Time: 5 minutes

Cooking Time: 10 minutes

Ingredients:

- Cauliflower rice: 2 cups
- Butter: 3 oz.
- Onion flakes: 3 teaspoon
- Pepper: ½ teaspoon
- Salt: ½ teaspoon
- Tomato puree: ¼ cup
- Cilantro -chopped finely: 2 teaspoons

Directions:

1. Melt the butter in a pan and sauté the onion flakes and garlic powder in it for 3 minutes.

2. Mix in the salt, pepper, and cauliflower rice, stir cook for another 3 minutes.

3. Mix in the tomato puree and cook for yet another 3 minutes.

4. Remove from the flame and mix in the cilantro.

Nutrition Value:

271 Cal, 23 g total fat -15 g sat. fat, 61 mg chol., 372 mg sodium, 12 g carbs, 5 g fiber, 5 g protein.

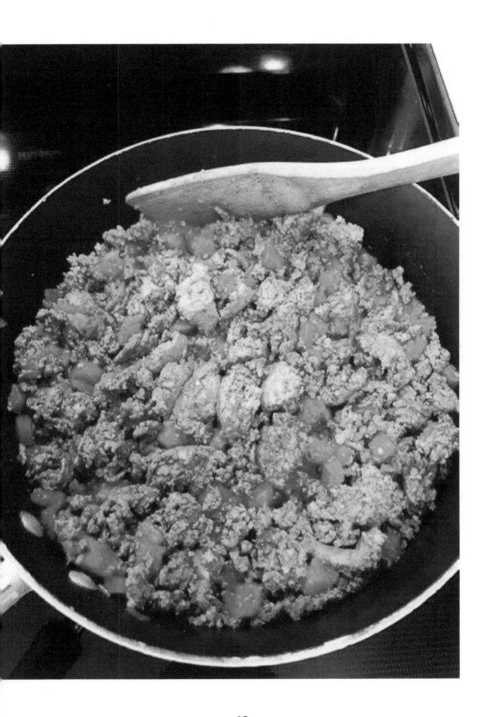

MEAT

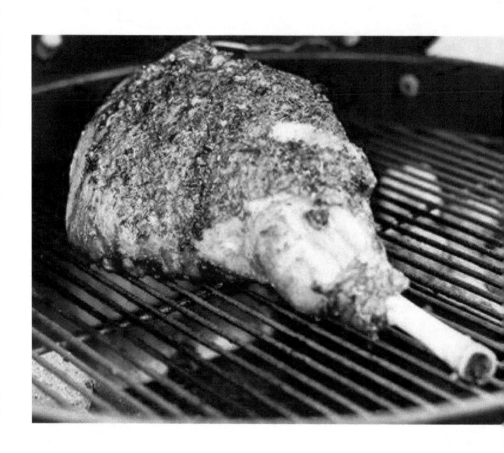

Shepherd's Pie

Preparation Time: 5 minutes

Cooking Time: 3-9 minutes

Servings: 2

Ingredients:

- 1/4 cup olive oil
- 1-pound grass-fed ground beef
- 1/2 cup celery, chopped
- 1/4 cup yellow onion, chopped
- 3 garlic cloves, minced
- cup tomatoes, chopped
- (12-ounce) packages riced cauliflower, cooked and well-drained
- 1 cup cheddar cheese, shredded
- 1/4 cup Parmesan cheese, shredded
- 1 cup heavy cream
- teaspoon dried thyme

Directions:

1. Preheat your oven to 350°F.
2. Heat oil heat and cook the ground beef, celery, onions, and garlic for about 8–10 minutes.
3. Immediately stir in the tomatoes.
4. Transfer mixture into a 10x7-inch casserole dish evenly.

5. In a food processor, add the cauliflower, cheeses, cream, thyme, and pulse until a mashed potatoes-like mixture is formed.

6. Spread the cauliflower mixture over the meat in the casserole dish evenly. Bake for about 35–40 minutes.

7. Cut into desired sized pieces and serve.

Nutrition:

Calories: 387 Fat: 11.5g Fiber: 9.4g Carbohydrates: 5.5 g Protein: 18.5g

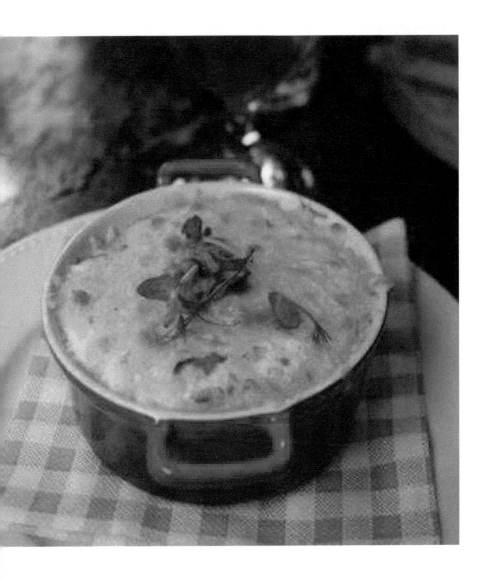

Beef Chili

Preparation Time: 10 minutes

Cooking Time: 50 minutes

Servings: 4

Ingredients:

- 1/2 green bell pepper, cored, seeded, and chopped
- 1/2 medium onion, chopped
- tablespoons extra-virgin olive oil
- 1 tablespoon minced garlic
- 1-pound ground beef (80/20)
- 1 (14-ounce) can crushed tomatoes
- 1 cup beef broth
- 1 tablespoon ground cumin
- 1 tablespoon chili powder
- 2 teaspoons paprika
- 1 teaspoon pink Himalayan sea salt
- 1/4 teaspoon cayenne pepper

Directions:

1. In a medium pot, combine the bell pepper, onion, and olive oil. Cook over medium heat for 8 to 10 minutes until the onion is translucent. Add the garlic and sauté.

2. Add the ground beef and cook for 7 to 10 minutes, until browned.

3. Add the tomatoes, broth, cumin, chili powder, paprika, salt, and cayenne. Stir to combine.

4. Simmer the chili for 30 minutes, until the flavors come together, then enjoy.

Nutrition:

Calories: 376 Fat: 18.4g Fiber: 12g Carbohydrates: 3.2 g Protein: 15.1g

Egg Roll Bowls

Preparation Time: 10minutes

Cooking Time: 30 minutes

Servings: 4

Ingredients:

- 1 tbsp. vegetable oil
- 1 clove garlic, minced
- 1 tbsp. minced fresh ginger
- 1 lb. ground pork
- 1 tbsp. sesame oil
- 1/2 onion, thinly sliced
- 1 c. shredded carrot
- 1/4 green cabbage, thinly sliced
- 1/4 c. soy sauce
- 1 tbsp. Sriracha
- green onion, thinly sliced
- 1 tbsp. sesame seeds

Directions:

1. Heat oil.

2. Put garlic and ginger and cook until fragrant, about 1 to 2 minutes. Put pork and cook until no pink remains.

3. Push pork to the side and add sesame oil.

4. Put onion, carrot, and cabbage. Stir to combine with meat. Then put soy sauce and Sriracha.

5. Stir and cook until cabbage is tender, about 6 to 8 minutes. Move and mixture to a serving dish

6. Garnish with sesame seeds and green onions.

Nutrition:

Calories: 321 Fat: 15g Fiber: 9.5g Carbohydrates: 5.1 g Protein: 7.4g

Grilled Leg of Lamb

Servings: 10

Cooking Time: 30 minutes

Ingredients

- 1/3 cup olive oil
- ¼ cup fresh lemon juice
- 6 garlic cloves, chopped
- ½ cup fresh oregano, chopped
- Salt and ground black pepper, as required
- 1 4½-pounds grass-fed boneless leg of lamb, trimmed and butterflied

Directions:

1. In a shallow glass baking dish, mix well oil, lemon juice, garlic, oregano, salt, and black pepper.
2. Add the leg of lamb and generously coat with the mixture.
3. Cover the baking dish and refrigerate to marinate overnight, flipping occasionally.
4. Preheat the charcoal grill to medium-high heat. Grease the grill grate.
5. Remove the leg of lamb from the refrigerator.
6. Carefully, insert a long metal skewer crosswise in the butterflied leg.

7. Place leg of lamb onto the grill and cook for about 20-30 minutes, flipping occasionally.

8. Remove from oven and place the leg of lamb over a cutting board.

9. With a piece of foil, cover the leg loosely for about 5-10 minutes before slicing.

10. With a sharp knife, cut the leg of lamb into desired size slices and serve.

Nutrition Info (Per Serving): Calories: 452; Net Carbs: 1.5g; Carbohydrate: 3.1g; Fiber: 1.6g; Protein: 57.9g; Fat: 22.1g; Sugar: 0.3g; Sodium: 173mg

Herb-simmered Beef Stew

Servings: 6

Cooking Time: 55 minutes

Ingredients

- 2 teaspoons lard, at room temperature
- 1 ½ pounds top chuck, cut into bite-sized cubes
- 1 celery stalk, chopped
- 2 Italian peppers, chopped
- 1/2 cup onions, chopped
- Kosher salt, to season
- 1/4 teaspoon freshly cracked black pepper, to taste
- 2 ripe tomatoes, pureed
- 4 cups vegetable broth
- 1 sprig thyme
- 1 sprig rosemary
- 1 bay laurel
- 2 tablespoons fresh chives, roughly chopped

Directions:

1. Melt the lard in a soup pot over medium-high heat. Sear the top chuck cubes for 8 to 9 minutes until brown; reserve, keeping it warm.

2. Then, in the pan drippings, sauté the celery, Italian peppers, and onions for 5 minutes until they have softened. Add in

the garlic and continue to sauté for 30 seconds to 1 minute longer or until aromatic.

3. Add the reserved beef back to the pot along with the salt, black pepper, tomatoes, vegetable broth, thyme, rosemary, and bay laurel.

4. Bring to a boil and immediately turn the heat to medium-low. Allow it to cook, partially covered, for 35 minutes longer.

5. Garnish with fresh chives and serve in individual bowls. Bon appétit!

Nutrition Info (Per Serving): 277 Calories; 21.5g Fat; 2.7g Carbs; 17.4g Protein; 0.8g Fiber

Sweet & Sour Pork Chops

Servings: 6

Cooking Time: 50 minutes

Ingredients

- 6 8-ounces ¾-inch thick pork shoulder chops, trimmed
- Salt and ground black pepper, as required
- 2 tablespoons olive oil
- 1¼ cups water
- ¾ cup organic apple cider vinegar
- 6 garlic cloves, mashed
- 2 tablespoons Erythritol
- 2 tablespoons fresh parsley, minced

Directions:

1. Preheat the oven to 400 degrees F.

2. Season each chop evenly with salt and black pepper.

3. In a large Dutch oven, heat the oil over high heat and sear the chops in 2 batches for about 5 minutes, flipping once halfway through.

4. Remove the pan from heat and arrange the chops in a single layer.

5. In a bowl, add the remaining ingredients except for the parsley and mix well.

6. Add the vinegar mixture evenly over chops.

7. Cover the pan and transfer it into the oven.

8. Bake for about 40 minutes.

9. Garnish with parsley and serve hot.

Nutrition Info (Per Serving): Calories: 777; Net Carbs: 1.3g; Carbohydrate: 1.4g; Fiber: 0.1g; Protein: 51.2g; Fat: 61.1g; Sugar: 0.2g; Sodium: 189mg

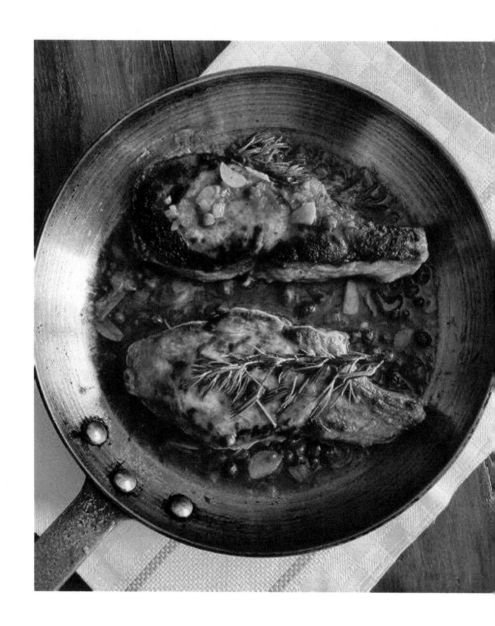

POULTRY

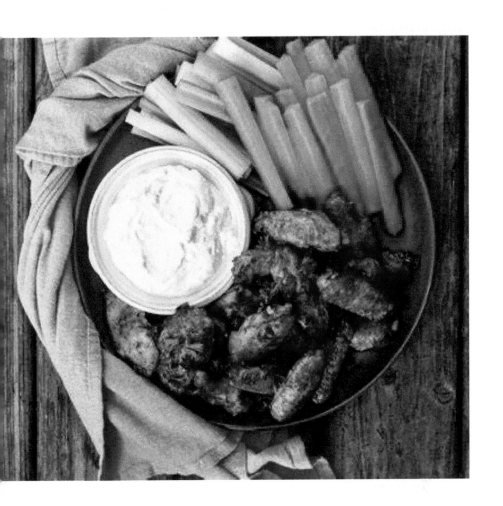

Chicken Breasts with Cheddar & Pepperoni

Servings: 4

Cooking Time: 40 minutes

Ingredients

- 12 oz canned tomato sauce
- 1 tbsp olive oil
- 4 chicken breast halves, skinless and boneless
- Salt and ground black pepper, to taste
- 1 tsp dried oregano
- 4 oz cheddar cheese, sliced
- 1 tsp garlic powder
- 2 oz pepperoni, sliced

Directions:

1. Preheat your oven to 390° F. In a bowl, combine chicken with oregano, salt, garlic, and pepper.

2. Heat a pan with the olive oil over medium heat, add in the chicken, cook each side for minutes, and remove to a baking dish. Top with the cheddar cheese slices, spread the sauce, then cover with pepperoni slices. Bake for 30 minutes. Serve warm garnished with fresh oregano if desired.

Nutrition Info (Per Serving): Kcal 387, Fat 21g, Net Carbs 4.5g, Protein 32g

Buffalo Spinach Chicken Sliders

Servings: 4

Cooking Time: 3 Hours 30 minutes

Ingredients

- 4 zero carb hamburger buns, halved
- 3 lb chicken thighs, boneless and skinless
- 1 tsp onion powder
- 2 tsp garlic powder
- Salt and black pepper to taste
- 2 tbsp ranch dressing mix
- ¼ cup white vinegar
- 2 tbsp hot sauce
- ½ cup chicken broth
- ¼ cup melted butter
- ¼ cup baby spinach
- 4 slices cheddar cheese

Directions:

1. In a bowl, combine onion and garlic powders, salt, pepper, and ranch dressing mix. Rub the mixture onto the chicken and place it into a pot; in another bowl, mix vinegar, hot sauce, broth, and butter.

2. Pour the mixture all over the chicken and cook on low heat for 3 hours.

3. Using two forks, shred the chicken into small strands. Mix and adjust the taste.

4. Divide the spinach in the bottom half of each low carb bun, spoon the chicken on top, and add a cheddar cheese slice. Cover with the remaining bun halves and serve.

Nutrition Info (Per Serving): Cal 774; Net Carbs 15.7g; Fat 37g; Protein 87g

Paprika Chicken Wings

Servings: 4

Cooking Time: 20 minutes

Ingredients

- 1 pound chicken wings
- 1 tablespoon cumin, ground
- 1 teaspoon coriander, ground
- 1 tablespoon sweet paprika
- A pinch of salt and black pepper
- 1 tablespoon lime juice
- 2 tablespoons olive oil

Directions:

1. In a bowl, mix the chicken wings with the cumin and the other ingredients, toss, spread them on a baking sheet lined with parchment paper and cook at 420 degrees F for 20 minutes.

2. Divide between plates and serve.

Nutrition Info: calories 286, fat 16, fiber 0.8, carbs 1.6, protein 33.3

Curry Chicken

Servings: 4

Cooking Time: 30 minutes

Ingredients

- 1 pound chicken breast, skinless, boneless and cubed
- 1 tablespoon olive oil
- 1 tablespoon yellow curry paste
- 1 cup chicken stock
- A pinch of salt and black pepper
- 1 teaspoon sweet paprika
- ½ teaspoon allspice, ground
- 1 tablespoon cilantro, chopped

Directions:

1. Heat up a pan with the oil over medium heat, add the meat and brown it for 5 minutes.
2. Add the curry paste and the other ingredients, toss, bring to a simmer and cook for minutes.
3. Divide the mix into bowls and serve.

Nutrition Info: calories 334, fat 24, fiber 2, carbs 4.5, protein 27

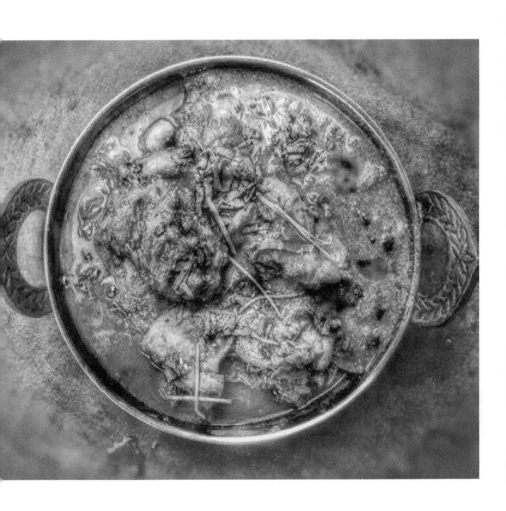

FISH

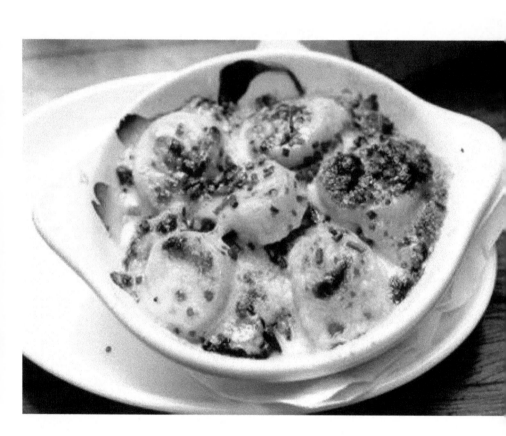

Lemony Sea Bass Fillet

Preparation Time: 10 minutes

Cooking Time: 10-15 minutes

Servings: 4

Ingredients:

Fish:

- 4 sea bass fillets
- 2 tablespoons olive oil, divided
- A pinch of chili pepper
- Salt, to taste

Olive Sauce:

- tablespoon green olives, pitted and sliced
- 1 lemon, juiced
- Salt, to taste

Directions:

1. Preheat the grill to high heat.

2. Stir together one tablespoon olive oil, chili pepper, and salt in a bowl. Brush both sides of each sea bass fillet generously with the mixture.

3. Grill the fillets on the preheated grill for about 5 to 6 minutes on each side until lightly browned.

4. Meanwhile, warm the left olive oil in a skillet over medium heat. Add the green olives, lemon juice, and salt.

5. Cook until the sauce is heated through.

6. Transfer the fillets to four serving plates, then pour the sauce over them. Serve warm.

Nutrition:

Calories: 257 Fat: 12.4g, Fiber: 56.g Carbohydrates: 2 g Protein: 12.7g

Curried Fish with Super Greens

Preparation Time: 10 minutes

Cooking Time: 20 minutes

Servings: 4

Ingredients:

- tablespoons coconut oil
- 2 teaspoons garlic, minced
- 11/2 tablespoons grated fresh ginger
- 1/2 teaspoon ground cumin
- 1 tablespoon curry powder
- 2 cups of coconut milk
- 16 ounces (454 g) firm white fish, cut into 1-inch chunks
- 1 cup kale, shredded
- 2 tablespoons cilantro, chopped

Directions:

1. Melt the coconut oil in a heated pan
2. Add the garlic and ginger and sauté for about 2 minutes until tender.
3. Fold in the cumin and curry powder, then cook for 1 to 2 minutes until fragrant.
4. Put in the coconut milk and boil. Boil, then simmer until the flavors mellow, about 5 minutes.

5. Add the fish chunks and simmer for 10 minutes until the fish flakes easily with a fork, stirring once.

6. Scatter the shredded kale and chopped cilantro over the fish, then cook for 2 minutes more until softened.

Nutrition:

Calories: 376 Fat: 19.9g Fiber: 15.8g, Carbohydrates: 6.7 g, Protein: 14.8 g

Shrimp Alfredo

Preparation Time: 15 minutes

Cooking Time: 30 minutes

Servings: 4

Ingredients:

- 1 pound of wild shrimp
- 3 tablespoons of organic grass-fed whey
- 1 1/2 cups of frozen asparagus
- a cup of heavy cream
- 1/2 cup of parmesan cheese
- Sea salt
- Black pepper
- ground garlic cloves
- 1 small diced onion

Directions:

1. Peel and devein the shrimps, coat them well with salt and pepper. Let it cover
2. in a bowl for 20 minutes.
3. Preheat a skillet. Put in butter, garlic, and onions.
4. When butter is melted, put in shrimp and stir fry till for 3 minutes.
5. Pour in heavy cream and stir well. Then, add ion cheese and stir till cheese melts.
6. Serve hot.

Nutrition:

Calories: 315, Fat: 11.9g Fiber: 8.5g, Carbohydrates: 9.3 g Protein: 11.1g

Garlic-Lemon Mahi Mahi

Preparation Time: 15 minutes

Cooking Time: 10 minutes

Servings: 3

Ingredients:

- 6 tablespoons of butter
- 5 tablespoons of extra-virgin olive oil
- 4 ounces of mahi-mahi fillets
- 3 minced cloves of garlic
- Kosher salt
- Black pepper
- 2 pounds of asparagus
- 2 sliced lemons
- Zest and juice of 2 lemons
- 1 teaspoon of crushed red pepper flakes
- 1 tablespoon of chopped parsley

Directions:

1. Melt three tablespoons of butter and olive oil in a microwave.

2. Heat a skillet and put in mahi-mahi, then sprinkle black pepper.

3. For around 5 minutes per side, cook it. When done, move to a plate.

4. In another skillet, add remaining oil and add in the asparagus, stir fry for 2-3 minutes. Take out on a plate.

5. In the same skillet, pour in the remaining butter, and add garlic, red pepper, lemon, zest, juice, and parsley.

6. Add in the mahi-mahi and asparagus and stir together. Serve hot.

Nutrition:

Calories: 317 Fat: 8.5g Fiber: 6.9g, Carbohydrates: 3.1 g Protein: 16.1g

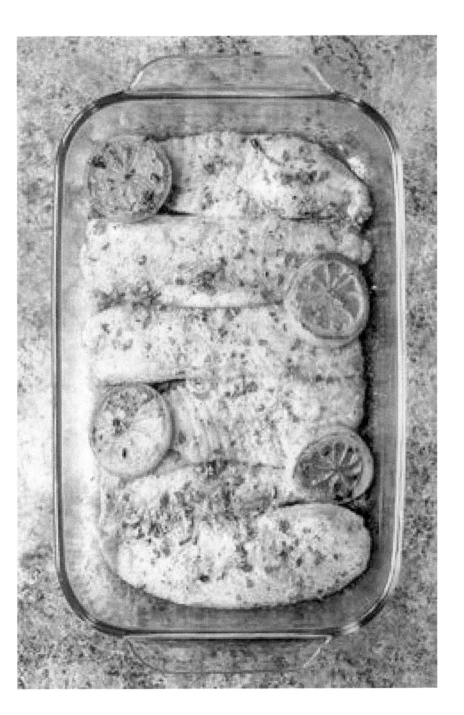

Scallops in Creamy Garlic Sauce

Preparation Time: 15 minutes

Cooking Time: 15 minutes

Servings: 4

Ingredients:

- 11/4 pounds fresh sea scallops, side muscles removed
- Salt and ground black pepper, as required
- 4 tablespoons butter, divided
- 5 garlic cloves, chopped
- 1/4 cup homemade chicken broth
- 1 cup heavy cream
- tablespoon fresh lemon juice
- tablespoons fresh parsley, chopped

Directions:

1. Sprinkle the scallops evenly with salt and black pepper.

2. Melt two tablespoons of butter in a large pan over medium-high heat and cook the scallops for about 2–3 minutes per side.

3. Flip the scallops and cook for about two more minutes. With a slotted spoon, transfer the scallops onto a plate.

4. Using the same pan, the butter must be melted and sauté the garlic for about 1 minute.

5. Pour the broth and bring to a gentle boil. Cook for about 2 minutes.

6. Stir in the cream and cook for about 1–2 minutes or until slightly thickened. Stir in the cooked scallops and lemon juice and remove from heat.

7. Garnish with fresh parsley and serve hot.

Nutrition:

Calories: 259 Fat: 8.5g Fiber: 7.4g, Carbohydrates: 2.1 g Protein: 12.2g

Shrimp Curry

Preparation Time: 15 minutes

Cooking Time: 20 minutes

Servings: 4

Ingredients:

- 2 tablespoons coconut oil
- 1/2 of yellow onion, minced
- 2 garlic cloves, minced
- 1 teaspoon ground turmeric
- 1 teaspoon ground cumin
- 1 teaspoon paprika
- 1 (14-ounce) can unsweetened coconut milk
- 1 large tomato, chopped finely
- Salt, as required
- 1-pound shrimp, peeled and deveined
- 2 tablespoons fresh cilantro, chopped

Directions:

1. The coconut oil must be melted in a wok on medium heat and sauté the onion for about 5 minutes.

2. Add the garlic and spices, and sauté for about 1 minute.

3. Add the coconut milk, tomato, and salt, and bring to a gentle boil. Let the curry simmer for about 10 minutes, stirring occasionally. Stir in the shrimp and cilantro and simmer for about 4–5 minutes.

Nutrition:

Calories: 354, Fat: 12.5g Fiber: 7.5 g, Carbohydrates: 4.1 g Protein: 14.1g

Israeli Salmon Salad

Preparation Time: 10 minutes

Cooking Time: 0 minutes

Servings: 2

Ingredients:

- 1 cup flaked smoked salmon
- 1 tomato, chopped
- 1/2 small red onion, chopped
- 1 cucumber, chopped
- 6 tbsp. pitted green olives
- 1 avocado, chopped
- 2 tbsp. avocado oil
- 2 tbsp. almond oil
- 1 tbsp. plain vinegar
- Salt and black pepper to taste
- 1 cup crumbled feta cheese
- 1 cup grated cheddar cheese

Directions:

1. In a salad bowl, add the salmon, tomatoes, red onion, cucumber, green olives, and avocado. Mix well.

2. In a bowl, whisk the avocado oil, vinegar, salt, and black pepper. Drizzle the dressing over the salad and toss well.

3. Sprinkle some feta cheese and serve the salad immediately.

Nutrition:

Calories: 415 Fat: 11.4g Fiber: 9.9g, Carbohydrates: 3.8 g Protein: 15.4g

VEGETABLES

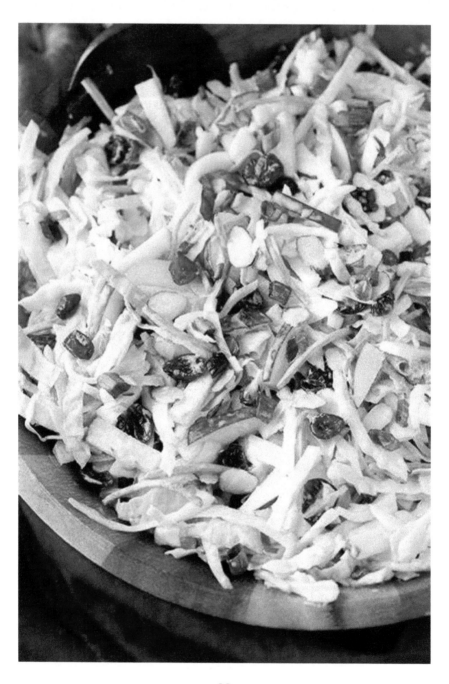

Tofu Sesame Skewers with Warm Kale Salad

Preparation Time: 2 hrs.

Cooking Time: 25 minutes

Servings: 4

Ingredients:

- 14 oz Firm tofu
- 4 tsp. sesame oil
- 1 lemon, juiced
- 5 tbsp. sugar-free soy sauce
- tsp. garlic powder
- 4 tbsp. coconut flour
- 1/2 cup sesame seeds

Warm Kale Salad:

- cups chopped kale
- 2 tsp. + 2 tsp. olive oil
- 1 white onion, thinly sliced
- 3 cloves garlic, minced
- 1 cup sliced white mushrooms
- 1 tsp. chopped rosemary
- Salt and black pepper to season
- tbsp. balsamic vinegar

Directions:

1. In a bowl, mix sesame oil, lemon juice, soy sauce, garlic powder, and coconut flour.

2. Wrap the tofu in a paper towel, squeeze out as much liquid from it, and cut it into strips.

3. Stick on the skewers, height-wise.

4. Place onto a plate, pour the soy sauce mixture over, and turn in the sauce to be adequately coated.

5. Heat the griddle pan over high heat.

6. Pour the sesame seeds on a plate and roll the tofu skewers in the seeds for a generous coat.

7. Grill the tofu in the griddle pan to be golden brown on both sides, about 12 minutes.

8. Heat 2 tablespoons of olive oil in a skillet over medium heat and sauté onion to begin browning for 10 minutes with continuous stirring.

9. Add the remaining olive oil and mushrooms.

10. Continue cooking for 10 minutes. Add garlic, rosemary, salt, pepper, and balsamic vinegar.

11. Cook for 1 minute.

12. Put the kale in a salad bowl; when the onion mixture is ready, pour it on the kale and toss well.

13. Serve the tofu skewers with the warm kale salad and a peanut butter dipping sauce.

Nutrition:

Calories: 276 Fat: 11.9g Fiber: 9.4g Carbohydrates: 21 g Protein: 10.3g

Cheesy Stuffed Peppers

Preparation Time: 15 minutes

Cooking Time: 40 minutes

Servings: 4

Ingredients:

- 2 tbsp. olive oil
- 4 red bell peppers, halved and seeded
- 1 cup ricotta cheese
- 1/2 cup gorgonzola cheese, crumbled
- 2 cloves garlic, minced
- 1 1/2 cups tomatoes, chopped
- 1 tsp. dried basil
- Salt and black pepper, to taste
- 1/2 tsp. oregano

Directions:

1. Let the oven heat up to 350° F.

2. In a bowl, mix garlic, tomatoes, gorgonzola, and ricotta cheeses.

3. Stuff the pepper halves and remove them to the baking dish. Season with oregano, salt, cayenne pepper, black pepper, and basil.

Nutrition:

Calories: 295 Fat: 12.4g Fiber: 10.1g Carbohydrates: 5.4 g Protein: 13.2g

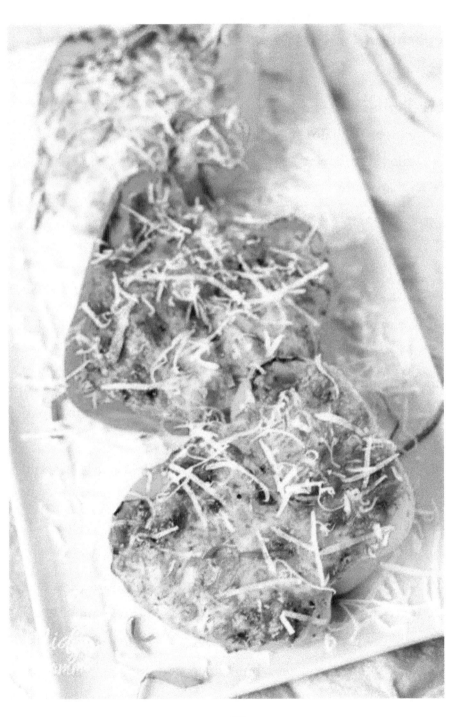

Easy-to-Prepare Broccoli

Preparation Time: 15 minutes

Servings: 4

Ingredients:

- cups broccoli florets
- minced garlic cloves
- 1 tbsp. butter
- 1 tbsp. fresh lime juice
- Salt, to taste

Directions:

1. In the bottom of the Instant Pot, arrange a steamer basket and pour 1 cup of water.
2. Place the broccoli into the steamer basket.
3. Secure the lid and place the pressure valve in the "Seal" position.
4. Select "Manual" and cook under "Low Pressure" for about 10 minutes.
5. Select the "Cancel" and carefully do a "Natural" release.
6. Remove the lid and transfer the broccoli to a plate.
7. Remove water from the pot and with paper towels, pat dry.
8. Place the butter in the Instant Pot and select "Sauté." Then add the garlic and cook for about 30 seconds.
9. Add the broccoli and lime juice and cook for about 30 seconds.

10. Stir in salt and cook for about 1 minute.

11. Select the "Cancel" and serve.

Nutrition Values:

Calories 64, Total Fat 3.2g, Net Carbs 1.9g, Protein 2.9g, Fiber 2.5g

Squid Salad with Mint, Cucumber & Chili Dressing

Servings: 4

Cooking Time: 30 minutes

Ingredients

- 4 medium squid tubes, cut into strips
- ½ cup mint leaves
- 2 medium cucumbers, halved and cut in strips
- ½ cup coriander leaves, reserve the stems
- ½ red onion, finely sliced
- Salt and black pepper to taste
- 1 tsp fish sauce
- 1 red chili, roughly chopped
- 1 clove garlic
- 2 limes, juiced
- 1 tbsp chopped coriander
- 1 tsp olive oil

Directions:

1. In a salad bowl, mix mint leaves, cucumber strips, coriander leaves, and red onion. Season with salt, black pepper and some olive oil; set aside. In the mortar, pound the coriander stems and red chili to form a paste using the pestle. Add the fish sauce, lime juice, and mix with the pestle.

2. Heat a skillet over high heat on a stovetop and sear the squid on both sides to lightly brown, about 5 minutes. Pour the squid on the salad and drizzle with the chili dressing. Toss the ingredients with two spoons, garnish with coriander, and serve the salad as a single dish or with some more seafood.

Nutrition Info (Per Serving): Kcal 318, Fat 22.5g, Net Carbs 2.1g, Protein 24.6g

Family Coleslaw with Cauliflower

Servings: 5

Cooking Time: 15 minutes

Ingredients

- 1 cup green cabbage, shredded
- 1 cup fresh cauliflower, chopped
- 4 tablespoons shallots, chopped
- 1 teaspoon garlic, minced
- 1 teaspoon lime juice
- 1 teaspoon white wine vinegar
- 1/3 cup mayonnaise
- Sea salt and ground black pepper, to taste

Directions:

1. Add the cabbage, cauliflower, shallots, and garlic to a salad bowl.

2. In a small mixing dish, whisk the lime juice, vinegar, mayonnaise, salt, and pepper.

3. Dress the salad and serve immediately. Bon appétit!

Nutrition Info (Per Serving): 121 Calories; 8.5g Fat; 6.8g Carbs; 3.3g Protein; 2.3g Fiber

DESSERT

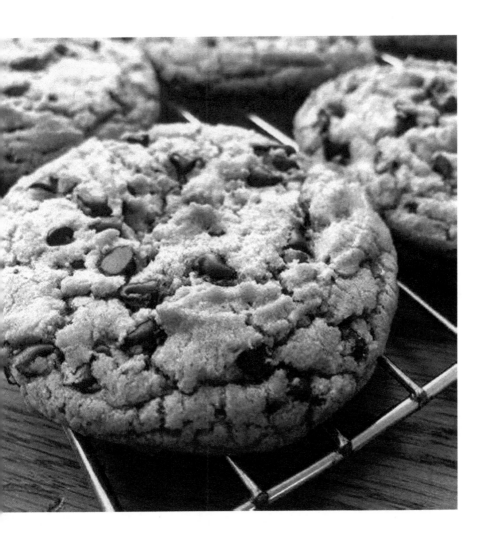

Red Berries Fat Bombs

Servings: 4

Cooking Time: 20 minutes

Ingredients

- 1 cup strawberries
- 1 cup raspberries
- 1 cup cranberries
- 1 tsp vanilla extract
- 16 oz cream cheese, softened
- 4 tbsp unsalted butter
- 2 tbsp sugar-free maple syrup

Directions:

1. Line a muffin tray with liners and set aside.

2. Puree the fruits in a blender with the vanilla. In a saucepan, melt cream cheese and butter together over medium heat until mixed.

3. In a bowl, combine the fruit, cheese mixtures, and maple syrup evenly and fill the muffin tray with the mix. Refrigerate for 40 minutes and serve.

Nutrition Info (Per Serving): Cal 227, Net Carbs 3.1g, Fat 15g, Protein 4g

Walnut Chocolate Squares

Servings: 6

Cooking Time: 10 minutes

Ingredients

- 3½ oz dairy-free dark chocolate
- 4 tbsp vegan butter
- 1 pinch salt
- ¼ cup walnut butter
- ½ tsp vanilla extract
- ¼ cup chopped walnuts

Directions:

1. Microwave chocolate and vegan butter for 2 minutes.

2. Remove and mix in salt, walnut butter, and vanilla extract. Grease a small baking sheet with cooking spray and line with parchment paper.

3. Pour in the batter and top with walnuts and chill in the refrigerator. Cut into squares.

Nutrition Info (Per Serving): Cal 125; Net Carbs 3g; Fat 10g; Protein 2g

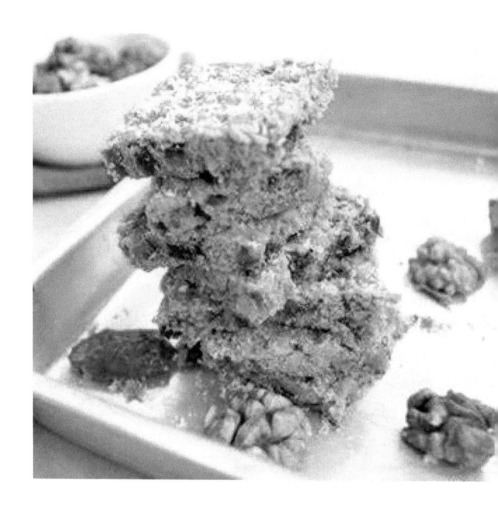

Speedy Custard Tart

Servings: 4

Cooking Time: 75 minutes

Ingredients

- ¼ cup butter, cold and crumbled
- ¼ cup almond flour
- 3 tbsp coconut flour
- ½ tsp salt
- 3 tbsp erythritol
- 1 ½ tsp vanilla extract
- 4 whole eggs
- 2 whole eggs + 3 egg yolks
- ½ cup swerve sugar
- 1 tsp vanilla bean paste
- 2 tbsp coconut flour
- 1 ¼ cup almond milk
- 1 ¼ cup heavy cream
- 2 tbsp sugar-free maple syrup
- ¼ cup chopped almonds

Directions:

1. Preheat oven to 350° F and grease a pie pan with cooking spray. In a bowl, mix almond flour, coconut flour, and salt. Add in butter and mix with an electric mixer until crumbly.

Add in erythritol and vanilla extract and mix. Pour in the four eggs one after another while mixing until formed into a ball.

2. Dust a clean flat surface with almond flour, unwrap the dough, roll out the dough into a large rectangle, fit into the pie pan; prick the crust base. Bake until golden. Remove after and allow cooling.

3. In a mixing bowl, whisk the whole eggs, 3 egg yolks, swerve sugar, vanilla bean paste, and coconut flour. Put the almond milk, heavy cream, and maple syrup into a pot and bring to a boil. Pour the mixture into the egg mixture and whisk while pouring. Run batter through a fine strainer into a bowl and skim off any froth. Remove the parchment paper, and transfer the egg batter into the pie. Bake for 45 minutes. Garnish with almonds, slice, and serve.

Nutrition Info (Per Serving): Cal 459; Net Carbs 1.2g, Fat 40g, Protein 12g

Greek-style Cheesecake

Servings: 6

Cooking Time: 1 Hour 35 minutes

Ingredients

- 2 cups almond meal
- 6 tablespoons butter, melted
- 1/2 teaspoon cinnamon
- 2 tablespoons Greek-style yogurt
- 10 ounces cream cheese softened
- 2 cups confectioner's Swerve
- 2 Eggs

Directions:

1. Mix the almond meal, butter, and cinnamon until well blended. Press the mixture into a parchment-lined baking pan. Then, whip the Greek-style yogurt, cream cheese, and confectioner's Swerve until well combined. Fold in the eggs, one at a time, and mix well after each addition.

2. Pour the filling over the crust in the baking pan. Bake in the preheated oven at 0 degrees F for about 30 minutes.

3. Run a sharp paring knife between the cheesecake and the baking pan and allow it to sit on the counter for 1 hour.

4. Cover loosely with plastic wrap and refrigerate overnight. Serve well-chilled and enjoy!

Nutrition Info (Per Serving): 471 Calories; 45g Fat; 6.9g Carbs; 11.5g Protein; 4g Fiber

Swiss Mascarpone Mousse with Chocolate

Servings: 6

Cooking Time: 15 minutes

Ingredients

For the mascarpone chocolate mousse:

- 8 oz mascarpone cheese
- 8 oz heavy cream
- 4 tbsp cocoa powder
- 4 tbsp xylitol

For the vanilla mousse:

- 3.5 oz cream cheese
- 3.5 oz heavy cream
- 1 tsp vanilla extract
- 2 tbsp xylitol

Directions:

1. In a bowl using an electric mixer, beat mascarpone cheese, heavy cream, cocoa, and xylitol until creamy. However, do not over mix. In another bowl, whisk all vanilla mousse ingredients until smooth and creamy. Gradually fold vanilla mousse mixture into the mascarpone one until well incorporated. Spoon into dessert cups and serve.

Nutrition Info (Per Serving): Cal 412; Net Carbs 5.9g; Fat 32g; Protein 8g

Almond Butter & Chocolate Cookies

Servings: 8

Cooking Time: 15 minutes

Ingredients

- 1 stick butter
- 1/2 cup almond butter
- 1/2 cup Monk fruit powder
- 3 cups pork rinds, crushed
- 1 teaspoon vanilla extract
- 1/4 teaspoon ground cinnamon
- 1/2 cup sugar-free chocolate, cut into chunks
- 1/2 cup double cream

Directions:

1. In a pan, melt the butter, almond butter, and Monk fruit powder over medium heat.

2. Now, add the crushed pork rinds and vanilla. Place the batter on a cookie sheet and let it cool in your refrigerator.

3. Meanwhile, in a small saucepan over medium heat, melt the chocolate and double cream. Add the chocolate layer over the batter.

4. Allow it to chill completely before slicing and serving. Bon appétit!

Nutrition Info (Per Serving):

322 Calories; 28.9g Fat; 3.4g Carbs; 0.6g Fiber; 13.9g Protein;